ROYAL COLLEGE OF PSYCHIATRISTS
ROYAL COLLEGE OF NURSING
BRITISH PSYCHOLOGICAL SOCIETY

Behaviour Modification

REPORT OF A JOINT WORKING PARTY
TO FORMULATE ETHICAL GUIDELINES
FOR THE CONDUCT OF PROGRAMMES OF
BEHAVIOUR MODIFICATION IN THE
NATIONAL HEALTH SERVICE

A CONSULTATIVE DOCUMENT WITH
SUGGESTED GUIDELINES

LONDON: HER MAJESTY'S STATIONERY OFFICE

ISBN 0 11 320732 8

FOREWORD

1.   As the opening paragraph of this report explains, it originated from a request made through one of my predecessors, Sir Keith Joseph, to the three professional bodies whose names are on its cover. This foreword gives me an opportunity of thanking them for their sponsorship and the members of the Working Party for their efforts.

2.   The task placed on these three bodies was a hard one. For the most difficult issues which have arisen in connection with behaviour modification programmes are those concerned with ethics and professional responsibility. It is intrinsic to the nature of professions that they must be watchful for their clients' interests, and they must still do so when the client himself has given his consent and put himself into the professional's hands. Behaviour modification programmes can raise difficult questions both as regards ends and as regards means. The guidance given in this report will, I am sure, be very valuable throughout the NHS, and indeed beyond it, to all those concerned with the carrying out of these programmes.

3.   The Working Party had to be a joint one, because the implementation of a behaviour modification programme is a joint task. If it cannot be undertaken with inter-professional agreement, the results could be less than satisfactory. Many people have pointed out that despite its many advantages, inter-professional teamwork has had the disadvantage that nobody quite knows what to do if the teamwork fails. There was no failure here. It is a tribute to the wisdom and patience of the Working Party members of the three professions—and to Professor Zangwill's chairmanship, that they were able to come to an agreement on some very difficult questions of professional working in what can be at times a controversial field.

4.   I have been asked to say that either Professor Zangwill as Chairman, or Mr Mellor as Secretary, will be glad to receive any comments on the guidelines.

5.   I hope that this well written and cogent report will be studied with the attention it deserves, to the benefit of all those involved in behaviour modification programmes.

Patrick Jenkin
Secretary of State for Social Services

MEMBERS OF THE WORKING PARTY

Professor O L Zangwill, MA FRS
Professor of Experimental Psychology, University of Cambridge (Chairman)

Professor D E Blackman, BA PhD FBPsS
Professor and Head of Department of Psychology, University College, Cardiff

Mrs J Dovey RMN SRN FPA
Nursing Officer, Regional Behaviour Research Unit, Hollymoor Hospital, Birmingham

Mr M Edwardes-Evans MA (Cantab)
Solicitor
Treasurer, National Association for Mental Health (MIND)

Mr J C Gardner, SRN RNMS DHSA
District Nursing Officer, North West District, Kensington and Chelsea and Westminster
Area Health Authority (Teaching)

Dr J N Hall BA MSc PhD
Principal Clinical Psychologist, Whitchurch Hospital, Cardiff

Dr W A Heaton-Ward MB ChB FRC Psych DPM
Consultant Psychiatrist, Stoke Park Hospital, Stapleton, Bristol
Clinical Teacher in Mental Health, University of Bristol

Mr M W Jackson RMNS SRN RMN Cert Beh Mod JBCNS
Nursing Officer, Lea Hospital, Bromsgrove

Dr C C Kiernan BA PhD
Deputy Director and Senior Research Officer, Thomas Coram Research Unit

Dr I S Kreeger MB BS FRC Psych DPM
Consultant Psychiatrist, King's College Hospital
Senior Tutor in Psychotherapy, Institute of Psychiatry, University of London

Mr F J Lewis
Senior Executive Officer, Department of Health and Social Security (Assistant
Secretary) (a)

Mr P D Mellor RMN RNMS
Nurse Adviser, Royal College of Nursing (Secretary)

Dr C P Seager MD FRC Psych
Senior Lecturer in Psychiatry, University of Sheffield

Miss P Whiffen Dip ASS
Social Work Education Adviser, Central Council for Education and Training in Social
Work (previously Assistant Director, National Association for Mental Health (MIND))

OBSERVERS

Mr S Moore
Principal Nursing Officer, Department of Health and Social Security

Dr R Wilkins
Principal Medical Officer, Department of Health and Social Security (b)

(a) Miss J A Vass, Higher Executive Officer, Department of Health and Social
Security, succeeded Mr Lewis from September 1977.

(b) Dr M J MacCulloch, Principal Medical Officer, Department of Health and
Social Security, succeeded Dr Wilkins as observer from May 1978.

CONTENTS

PREFACE

The Working Party's Report was originally submitted to the three parent bodies, viz the Royal College of Psychiatrists, the Royal College of Nursing and the British Psychological Society, for their approval. In response, a number of comments were received, and the Working Party reconvened to consider these comments. Some changes have been made to the Report. This is now the final Report.

Chapter 1
INTRODUCTION

1.   This Working Party was established as a consequence of the Department of Health and Social Security's response to the report* of a Professional Investigation into Medical and Nursing Practices on certain wards in Napsbury Hospital near St Albans, published in 1973. As the Investigating Team concluded that difficulties similar to those that arose at Napsbury Hospital might arise in relation to other programmes of behaviour modification which they believed were being introduced increasingly into NHS Hospitals, they recommended that the Department of Health and Social Security should consider the desirability of asking the Royal College of Psychiatrists, the Royal College of Nursing and the British Psychological Society to set up a joint working party to formulate ethical guidelines for the conduct of such programmes. (Napsbury Report, para 55).†

2.   These three bodies were duly approached by the Department of Health and Social Security and expressed their willingness to co-operate in setting up the proposed Working Party. Each parent body nominated four members to serve on it and one of the nominees of the British Psychological Society, Professor O L Zangwill, was invited to act as Chairman. To represent the "consumer interest", the Chairman invited the National Association for Mental Health (MIND), to nominate two lay members to join the Working Party. This the Association agreed to do.

3.   At its first meeting on 12 March 1974, the Chairman advised the Working Party that no formal terms of reference had been given him by the Department of Health and Social Security, who were content to let the Working Party decide their terms of reference for themselves in the light of Paragraph 55 of the Napsbury Report. The Working Party noted that programmes of behaviour modification were being introduced increasingly both inside and outside the National Health Service and that the professional organisations most closely concerned were being frequently asked for guidance on how these programmes should be implemented in order to avoid difficulties of the kind that had arisen at Napsbury Hospital.

4.   It was pointed out that the term "behaviour modification" itself gave rise to difficulty since it was open to varied interpretations. Members of the Working Party who had themselves been active in this field did not consider that the form of treatment at Napsbury Hospital was behaviour modification in the sense in which the term is understood by the majority of those at present engaged professionally in it. At the same time, the Working Party was in agreement with the view of the Professional Investigating Team that behaviour modification in the latter sense may give rise to difficulties similar to those to

---

*Published by HMSO 1973.

†The British Psychological Society has since set up its own Working Party on behaviour modification which has recently issued its report. Ethical considerations are briefly discussed on p 21 of the Report. (*Report of the Working Party on Behaviour Modification*. British Psychological Society, St Andrews House, 48 Princess Road East, Leicester LE1 7DR).

which attention had been directed in their Report. These difficulties were first, an undue inflexibility in implementing the programme such that there was "at times a seeming lack of compassion and of respect of the rights of patients" (Report, para 50); secondly, a failure adequately to instruct patients and their relations in the nature and aims of the treatment method, which might involve "complex reasoning which neither might be able to understand". (loc cit); and thirdly, production of anxiety and tension among the staff of the hospital, particularly in those not directly involved in the programme. The Investigating Team were therefore led to conclude that ". . . although their theoretical basis may have been unexceptionable, it is our opinion that the practical application of these methods in certain wards of Napsbury Hospital did lead to situations which should not exist in an NHS Hospital" (loc cit).

5.   As envisaged by the Working Party, the term *behaviour modification* refers to programmes in which attempts are made to apply to practical issues of management and treatment principles and techniques which have been developed in systematic experimental studies of human and animal behaviour (see Appendix I). At the same time, it is important to bear in mind that the content of a behaviour modification programme is never solely determined by scientific principles and techniques but must always relate to the particular type of behaviour disorder which it is designed to ameliorate and the particular objective which it is hoped to attain. It is in regard to these latter aspects, especially, that ethical issues are liable to obtrude.

6.   It should be pointed out that the term *behaviour modification* is commonly used to denote two different, if closely related, therapeutic approaches. In the first, commonly referred to as *behaviour therapy*, the emphasis is upon individual treatment and finds its main application in the treatment of psychoneurotic behaviour disorders. In the second, the emphasis is primarily upon group treatment, the aim being to modify aberrant behaviour in the individual through participation in the planned activity of an organised group. This second approach, which finds its main application in the treatment of mentally handicapped or chronic psychiatric patients, was accepted by the Working Party as its principal concern. The groups concerned are of varying size and may on occasion involve whole wards and units in hospitals and kindred institutions. It should be appreciated, however, that this form of behaviour modification is practised not only in the context of psychiatric medicine in institutions within the National Health Service but also in a number of other institutions, eg schools and prisons. There is even a sense in which it may be said to take place in the family and indeed in society generally. Because the Working Party was given its remit by the Department of Health and Social Security, it was felt that our discussions and recommendations should be couched predominantly in terms of clinical practice. None the less, we believe that a number of the issues considered and the recommendations made have direct relevance to bodies other than the Department of Health and Social Security.

7.   All matters pertaining to ethics inevitably raise grave difficulties of definition. While it is obviously difficult, if not impossible, to specify absolute criteria of ethical conduct, the Working Party was guided in its deliberations by traditional ethical standards of conduct in the medical, nursing and allied professions. By and large, these standards prescribe conduct that is generally accepted as humane, socially acceptable and, in so far as can be judged, in the

best interests of the individual patient. In so far as behaviour modification may entail subjective judgements as to the propriety of altering particular patterns of behaviour, the question of social acceptability is clearly of great importance. For this reason, the Working Party paid particular attention to ways in which behaviour modification procedures might appear *prima facie* liable to abuse and to ways in which they might be so adapted as to render them socially acceptable in the present climate of opinion.

8. In attempting to formulate guidelines, the Working Party felt strongly that their recommendations should be relevant to *any* attempt to modify behaviour whether or not it complied with the relatively strict definition of this term which the Working Party had agreed to accept (cf para 5 and Appendix I). For example, certain procedures which might comply with this definition might none the less be ethically undesirable, eg the excessive use of coercion or the manipulation of cash or goods. Further, it was appreciated that the less scrupulous might try to evade any guidelines which might be proposed by referring to their programmes by some name other than behaviour modification. It was therefore decided to focus attention upon the procedures actually employed rather than upon any particular name or names whereby they might be known.

9. In preliminary consideration of the ethical problems involved in the practice of behaviour modification, six main areas of concern were pinpointed which the Working Party agreed would need to be covered. These areas were increasingly clarified in the course of investigation and discussion and constitute the main body of this report. They may be specified as follows:—

(i) *Information and Access:* As was remarked by the Investigating Team with reference to Napsbury Hospital, "...much unhappiness could have been avoided by a better programme of preparation and public relations" (Report, para 51). It was therefore thought essential to consider the extent to which programmes of behaviour modification should be public, ie that full information concerning the programme should be available to the patient and his relatives, as also to members of the staff of the institution other than those directly responsible for implementing it. Information to relatives is of crucial importance in cases in which the patient himself may not be fully capable of grasping the information imparted to him. This, of course, is closely related to the issue of meaningful consent to accept treatment and is dealt with in some detail in Chapter 3 of this Report.

(ii) *Consent:* From an ethical point of view, consent to accept a given treatment is valid only if it is seen as a contract between the therapist and the patient, recognising that in certain cases parents will be asked to provide consent for children and that some adult patients will be unable to give consent. As certain types of behaviour modification programmes may involve a rescheduling of professional care, food or money, which are the patient's by right, it would seem essential that the issue of consent by, or on behalf of, patients participating in a programme should demand particularly careful consideration.

(iii) *Control:* Certain aspects of behaviour modification have given rise to controversy. Concern has been expressed about the goals of behavioural programmes and also about certain of the methods used to attain these goals. Examination of such matters may serve to focus attention on similar issues that may arise, if in a less extreme or less obvious form, with methods of treatment other than behaviour modification.

(iv) *Responsibility:* The issue of responsibility in the context of behaviour modification programmes poses particular problems in so far as non-medical personnel (eg clinical psychologists and nurses) no less than medical may be intimately involved in their design and conduct. Indeed many such programmes may be viewed as exercises in team work in which it is not always easy to specify precisely where professional responsibility primarily resides or in whom overall responsibility for the entire venture is vested.

(v) *Review Bodies:* In view of the fact that behaviour modification has social no less than medical aspects, the question of establishing Review Bodies to monitor and when necessary inspect behaviour modification programmes was thought to be a matter requiring careful consideration.

(vi) *Training:* In view of the multi-disciplinary character of behaviour modification and its recent introduction into British hospitals, the question of appropriate training for the design and implementation of behaviour modification programmes is clearly important. This question involves, if in somewhat different contexts, the training not only of psychiatrists, clinical psychologists and nursing staff, but of all other staff directly or indirectly involved, eg social workers, remedial teachers and occupational therapists, whether inside or outside the National Health Service.

10.   Having delineated these six closely inter-related themes, the Working Party set about obtaining such relevant information and evidence as bore on any or all of them. In the first instance, an attempt was made to ascertain the nature and scale of behaviour modification programmes at present being carried out in British psychiatric institutions. To this end, 526 hospitals in the United Kingdom, many of these being General Hospitals with few psychiatric beds, were approached in May 1974, and asked whether behaviour modification programmes were either projected or in progress. The 115 hospitals which responded positively to our inquiry, were again contacted and asked to provide information on various aspects of the programmes being undertaken. About three-quarters of these 115 hospitals gave us useful information, including evidence as to type of programme, number and kind of psychiatric patients involved, number and designation of staff attached to the particular programme, and details of staff training and the facilities made for contact with relatives and voluntary workers.

11.   This questionnaire disclosed that over half the 115 hospitals which responded mentioned that they used behaviour therapy with psychiatric patients, and a quarter of the responding hospitals mentioned that they employed various types of group programmes, for the most part involving chronic patients. Token economy techniques, which are perhaps the best known methods of modifying behaviour, were mentioned in the replies of about two-fifths of the hospitals. (These techniques are briefly described in Appendix I). A notable feature of the replies from mental handicap hospitals was the number of different programmes—up to seven—which might be in operation at any one time.

12.   Written evidence was sought from seventeen professional and other bodies concerned directly or indirectly with the care, treatment and

rehabilitation of psychiatric patients. Unsolicited material was submitted by certain other indviduals and bodies. These sources are listed in Appendices III and V.

13. In April 1975, members of the Committee (as a rule in groups of two or more) paid visits to a number of Mental Illness and Mental Handicap Hospitals at which it was known that behaviour modification programmes were, or had recently been, in active operation. These institutions are listed in Appendix IV. Reports on the visits were prepared by members of the Working Party and reviewed and discussed at full meetings of the Working Party.

14. The experience gained from these visits indicated that programmes of behaviour modification appear to have developed in a distinctly haphazard way and that the relative degree of involvement of different professional groups (psychiatrists, nurses, psychologists and medical auxiliary staff) varies widely from one institution to another. Practice as regards the obtaining of consent to treatment, involvement of relatives and assessment of results is likewise far from uniform and the allocation of responsibility within a behaviour modification team is sometimes far from clear. On several occasions, our attention was called to lack of overall planning and to severe deficiencies in training in methods of behaviour modification, particularly among nurses. In certain cases, programmes of behaviour modification had to be discontinued owing to lack of cooperation on the part of relatives. None the less, a fair degree of satisfaction with the outcome of behaviour modification programmes was frequently reported.

15. With regard to ethics, the view was commonly expressed that no distinctive ethical problems arise in connection with behaviour modification. However, we were informed that objections to the procedures used in certain programmes had been voiced on occasion by members of the staff of an institution (usually a nurse) or by the relatives of a patient who had taken part. Varying opinions were expressed as to the need for ethical guidelines but the Working Party gained the impression that they would be welcomed by many people actively engaged in the practice of behaviour modification. It was thought that the drawing up of guidelines would introduce greater uniformity in approach and lead to improved organisation and standards of training. Further, acceptable ethical guidelines might do much to clarify issues of responsibility, achieve the fuller co-operation of patients' relatives and reassure the public at large.

16. A certain number of individuals known to be interested in ethics in relation to psychiatric treatment were invited to meet the Working Party to discuss either general or more specific issues as might arise in connection with behaviour modification. These included philosophers and academic psychologists as well as psychiatrists, clinical psychologists and others known to be actively involved in the practice of behaviour modification. All but two of those invited were able to accept and provided the Working Party with a wide spectrum of views bearing on the six issues specified in paragraph 9 and related matters. The two who were invited but unable to attend submitted written statements. A list of the individuals who provided the Working Party with oral or written evidence is given in Appendix V.

Chapter 2
INFORMATION AND ACCESS

17.   Programmes of behaviour modification may involve procedures which appear novel, strange or even cruel to many not directly involved or trained in the implementation of such programmes. In their Report on the Napsbury case, the Professional Investigating Team comment that "The ideas may have been good ones but little appears to have been done to prepare patients, relatives, or staff in other parts of the hospital for policies which clearly were to cut right across traditional attitudes of medical and nursing care. It is our belief that the anxieties, anger and criticism which these new policies provoked, could have been foreseen, at least to some degree, and better public relations could have done much to prevent them. From talking to relatives we were convinced that some of them had not understood the reasons for these policies, which they genuinely felt to be cruel, unjust or even outrageous, and we could not but feel sympathy for their point of view". (Report, Paragraph 37). In consequence, they were led to conclude that "much unhappiness could have been avoided by a better programme of preparation and public relations". (Report, Paragraph 51).

18.   It would seem, therefore, that behaviour modification programmes must be public in the sense that full information concerning the treatment—the methods, objectives, expected progress and any major drawbacks—should be available to the patient and to relatives responsible for him, more especially in cases in which he may not be capable of fully understanding this information, before the programme is set in train. In our view, this should include a straightforward account of the general principles and objectives of behaviour modification as well as clear information relating to the particular treatment programme which is being proposed. Unless proper explanation is given, the hazard arises that relatives and friends may unwittingly frustrate the objectives of the programme, eg by gifts which in effect provide a "reward" which the patient has done nothing to earn. Even greater difficulty may arise if there is actual lack of cooperation on the part of relatives and others in carrying through a programme, even where initial cooperation was forthcoming. In our opinion, such a situation calls for even more detailed discussion with staff, patients and relatives in order to resolve mutual misunderstandings. All the evidence we received tended to confirm the view that lack of open discussion is counter-productive and potentially harmful.

19.   It is most important that information should also be given to the staff of any institution in which a programme of behaviour modification is instituted, even if such staff are not directly involved in its implementation. For those directly concerned, specific and detailed information regarding the methods, objectives and possible drawbacks of the programme should be given. For those not directly involved, general background information should be given before the programme is put into effect and should be followed up with ongoing information as to its progress. If possible, such information should reach all staff in the hospital or institution concerned. In short, there should be a full clinical discussion with all professional staff as well as detailed explanation to the patient, relatives and any others having a close relationship

with him. As a general rule it is important that the information given to both staff and patients or their relatives should enable behaviour modification to be seen, not as something special and separate, but as one of a number of treatment methods available. To this end, it might prove helpful if every hospital or institution concerned were to issue a leaflet giving information about behaviour modification in general and outlining the various behaviour modification programmes likely to be used.

20.   At the same time, it should be appreciated that cases may arise in which it might be thought undesirable to go into detail about a programme of behaviour modification specifically designed for a particular patient with staff other than those directly concerned with its conduct. Although this is most unlikely to arise with group behaviour modification programmes, it may well arise on occasion in connection with individual behaviour therapy, more especially if this should involve treatment for psychosexual disorders or other forms of deviance or the use of aversion therapy.

21.   Free access to all relevant information is of course necessary for informed *consent*. This should be envisaged not as a once and for all decision; ongoing and continuous explanation and opportunities for discussion should be included in the programme itself and viewed as an essential part of it. Otherwise, the concept of 'consent' has no real meaning. Issues relating to consent to treatment are further considered in Chapter 3.

22.   The provision of information relevant to behaviour modification should be subject to two conditions only. These are, first, the need for confidentiality; and secondly, the possibility that certain types of information may, if disseminated too widely, reduce therapeutic efficacy and so might be considered to be against the patient's own best interests. As regards confidentiality, it is obvious that patients should be protected from pressures, eg to appear on television or give interviews to the media. It may also be desirable to protect the feelings of parents and relatives from too widespread or detailed dissemination of information regarding a behaviour modification programme. In a wider setting, programmes of health education could well make reference to behaviour modification and explain and discuss what is meant and intended by such procedures.

23.   The Working Party is satisfied that only in exceptional cases should patients involved in any form of treatment be deprived of access by visitors and friends. This of course also includes treatment by behavioural methods, which it should be stressed by no means necessarily implies restrictions on access of any kind. Where, however, such restriction is considered to be in the patient's interest (ie determined by the design of a behaviour modification programme which it is genuinely thought will benefit him), it is essential that his consent should be forthcoming or, in cases in which it may be inappropriate, that of those others involved, ie relatives or staff. At the same time, any restrictions of access that are scheduled should be for specific reasons and within strict limits.

24.   It is important that the rights of privacy which all patients enjoy should be upheld. Visitors whose main object is mere curiosity about behaviour modification should therefore be discouraged, especially if the patient should feel that his privacy is being invaded. At the same time, undue isolation of patients in hospital is obviously undesirable and behaviour modification

should so far as possible be open to public scrutiny to allay anxiety or suspicion. Where there is conflict between this and the patient's right to privacy, the decision should rest not with the staff but with the person claiming such privacy, or where it is claimed on his behalf.

25. Regardless of any behaviour modification programme or other circumstances restricting access to patients, designated members of the appropriate Health Authority (Regional or Area Health Authority) should have unrestricted access, subject to the usual courtesies ie they should approach both the consultant in charge of the patient's treatment and the charge nurse of the ward prior to their visit to enable them to be present and discuss what was happening. So, also, should the members of any Review Committee as might be set up to approve and monitor behaviour modification programmes at Regional or Area Authority level. This matter is considered in Chapter 6.

26. A patient's nearest relatives should have unrestricted access except in cases in which a behaviour modification programme explicitly involves the manipulation of such access. In such cases, the considerations adduced in Paragraph 19 are particularly relevant and the Working Party consider that there is much to be said in favour of obtaining written consent from the patient and/or his nearest relatives before the programme is implemented. (See also Chapter 3, paragraph 31).

27. It is recommended that, whatever consents may have been obtained, no restriction should be placed on access for periods exceeding two weeks.

Chapter 3
CONSENT

28. In considering the ethics of any form of treatment practised in institutions for which the Department of Health and Social Security has responsibility, it is necessary to give more thought to those receiving the treatment than to those responsible for providing it. Insofar as consent marks the beginning of the treatment sequence, it is important to consider the process of obtaining that consent.

29. Consent is valid if it is seen as a contract between the person in charge of the treatment and the patient, recognising that parents will be asked to provide consent for children and that some adult patients will be unable to give consent.

30. Such a contract must be understood by those who are party to it. As pointed out in Paragraph 18, this entails explanations and acceptance of the goals of the treatment programme and of the methods used to attain these goals. While it would not be in the interest of the patient to require such specific forms of consent that the therapist could not make minor adjustments to his programme, the patient or other consenting party should be given a basic explanation of the targets, of potential disadvantages set against anticipated benefits, and of the methods, particularly where these are experimental or involve short-term pain or discomfort.

16

31.   The Working Party are unanimously of the view that no patient should ever be deprived of professional care. The practice of behaviour modification may, however, at times involve *rescheduling* or *restricting* the patient's access to food or money, curtailing visits or leave, the use of isolation or physical restraint, or cause him to experience a degree of discomfort. In such cases, the person in charge of the treatment may consider that written consent should be obtained in order to avoid any subsequent dispute as to what had been agreed. If such a procedure is followed, many patients for whom behaviour modification is the treatment of choice should be able to enter into a contract for their own treatment with full understanding and commitment.

32.   Consent is a continuous process so that substantial changes in the main targets or methods of a behaviour modification programme entail a renegotiation between therapist and patient or those consenting on his behalf.

33.   Some informal patients may wish to withdraw consent and to discontinue their treatment. They should be able to do so without absenting themselves and thereby prejudicing their chance of having an alternative, though not necessarily better, form of treatment.

34.   Behaviour modification programmes in an important sense involve the patient's total environment. Even where valid consent by adults is available, therefore, it is most important to involve relatives by providing the kind of information and explanation outlined in Paragraph 18 and thus helping them to understand the nature of the contract. Any objections raised by relatives should be treated sympathetically but should not interfere with a course of behaviour modification to which a patient has given and continues to give, informed consent. If this arises, the help of a social worker may prove of great benefit.

35.   Some patients are unable themselves to give valid consent. In such cases, every effort should be made to ensure that those concerned, whether patients, relatives or guardians, do understand the issue as far as possible. Many children have concerned, responsible parents to give consent on their behalf but others, particularly in residential or long-term hospital care, have an agency 'in loco parentis'. Where parental rights have been removed from the parents but may be restored, it would seem important that the social worker or others responsible should gain the parents' co-operation even though their consent may not be legally required.

36.   In law, no one has power to consent to treatment on behalf of any adult patient who is incapable of giving that consent. Nonetheless, the suggestion has been made that where a patient is incapable of giving consent, and where relatives are either unavailable or unable to take a decision, agreement might be sought either from an independent individual acting as a 'patient's friend' or 'third-party advocate', or from a Review Body (see Chapter 6).

37.   People in default of the law, whether in any form of legal detention or offered probation with conditions of residence and treatment, need special consideration. It is known that the use of behaviour modification methods generally throughout an institution has been proposed and this, if given effect, would raise special questions relevant to consent, more especially if alternative forms of treatment were not readily available. The validity of consent would be further prejudiced where the only choice available to the contracting

individual lay between prison and treatment by behaviour modification as a condition of probation.

38. We note that the Committee on Mentally Abnormal Offenders* has considered that there is some ambiguity about the position in the case of those compulsorily detained on treatment orders who have no right of appeal where particular forms of treatment (which may include behaviour modification) are proposed. This matter is also referred to in the consultative document on the review of the Mental Health Act†. We assume that the Department of Health and Social Security will be issuing advice on the subject and hence simply record our view that compulsorily detained patients should have some right of appeal where a programme of behaviour modification is proposed for them.

Chapter 4
CONTROL

39. In evidence submitted to this Working Party, it has been argued that it is unnecessary—even undesirable—to formulate ethical guidelines specifically for the conduct of behaviour modification programmes. It was contended that the ethical considerations that arise in this connection are no different from those arising with any other method of treatment or management of patients in psychiatric practice. On such a view, the only necessary guidelines are those common to good professional practice.

40. Even if this argument were accepted as a general statement, the Working Party felt that it failed to consider the possibility that different treatments might pose different ethical dilemmas, often of a very subtle kind. If definitive solutions to these dilemmas cannot always be found or agreed upon, setting out the ethical implications of certain treatment procedures may none the less help the people concerned in a practical capacity to make their own decisions.

41. Insofar as behaviour modification programmes involve social no less than therapeutic manipulations, they have given rise to understandable controversy. Concern has been expressed about the ethical propriety not only of the goals of some such programmes but also certain of the methods which have been used to achieve these goals. In this connection, it should be borne in mind that whereas the goals of behaviour modification may often be similar to those of other forms of treatment, the means by which it is sought to attain them (ie the techniques employed) are peculiar to behaviour modification. This distinction is not always clearly appreciated. Further, it should be added that any definition of what behaviour is 'desirable' and what 'undesirable' always presupposes a value judgement and may thus be highly controversial.

---

*CMND 6244
Published HMSO October 1975
†A Review of the Mental Health Act 1959
Published HMSO August 1976
(The White Paper "Review of the Mental Health Act 1959" has now been published—HMSO September 1978).

Goals of Treatment

42. In behaviour modification programmes, the practice of defining the desired outcome of treatment in precise behavioural terms has provided a stimulating challenge to clear thinking with regard to goals in psychiatric treatment generally. It throws into debate fundamental questions as to what indeed constitutes desirable behaviour and how decisions about such definitions are arrived at.

43. This is less obviously a matter of concern when it involves adults living at home, or who are capable of understanding the issues involved and of giving or withholding their consent. But it is clearly a matter of concern when it involves either children or mentally ill or mentally handicapped adults who are being treated in institutional settings. In such circumstances it is not simply a matter of obtaining appropriate consent. When an individual is totally dependent on the responses of others for care, sustenance and even freedom, a generally acceptable definition of desirable behaviour becomes crucial.

44. It is essential that the demands which are made on patients be appropriately related to their individual needs, abilities and capacity for change, growth and emotional development. At a more fundamental level, it is most important to recognise that all treatments concerned with changing behaviour are based on value judgements. The definition of desirable behaviour is relative. It is likely to vary in accordance with the ideology implicit in the aim of the treatment. For example, the expectation of the staff in Units managing patients simply by custodial care will be very different from those of staff in Units with active rehabilitation programmes. In the same way, the passive, cooperative attitudes appreciated by staff in general medical wards will differ markedly from the autonomy, initiative and responsibility expected of psychiatric patients in "therapeutic communities". Great care is needed if the individual's cultural values are to be respected and safeguarded against the unrecognised impositions of the values of the therapist or of the institution. When, for example, is one teaching patients adaptive skills and when is one moulding them into social conformity?

45. Hence the need arises to consider whether the goals decided upon are concerned primarily with the needs of the patient or with the convenience of the staff. These need not be in conflict but this should not be taken for granted. Such questions might arise, for example, as a result of teaching self-care behaviour in a token economy programme. A precedent, perhaps, exists in the history of the care of children admitted to hospital for investigation and treatment of physical illness. For long, parents were often discouraged from visiting because it "upset" the children when they left and, indeed, they seemed to "settle down" when the visits ceased. It was not until the work of John Bowlby and others led to the recognition of the psychological damage that may be done to young children by what appeared to them the permanent disappearance of their parents that the attitude towards visiting was completely reversed. In general, parents are now encouraged to spend as much time as possible at the hospital and there are nowadays even facilities for mothers to be admitted with the very small child who has to undergo surgery. This may seem self-evidently the right way to handle distress in children separated from their mothers but for long it failed to be appreciated owing to an unrecognised identification of the goals of treatment with the convenience of staff.

Basic Rights or Earned Privileges

46.   Ethical questions have arisen in connection with behaviour modification programmes which use rewards for behavioural change by manipulation of available material goods, activities and events, making them contingent upon appropriate behaviour. This has raised important questions about what the basic rights of patients should be and whether, if ever, they should be subordinated to the requirements of a behaviour modification programme.

47.   It is desirable, though not always possible, that all patients in institutional settings should have the basic right to expect a high standard of professional care; concerned and individual attention; a nutritionally adequate, attractive and varied diet; warm, comfortable accommodation; and the provision if needed of appropriate and attractive clothing. They should have the right to retain their own goods and money, eg pensions and social security benefits, subject to certain statutory regulations (Cf HM (71) 90) and the rules and regulations of the institutions in which they reside. They should have opportunities for recreational facilities as well as access to visitors and occupation.

48.   There is considerable evidence indicating that an impoverished environment is of itself a cause of disturbed behaviour. At the present time, it has to be recognised that despite prolonged endeavour, in many areas the basic rights referred to in the previous paragraph barely reach acceptable standards. In institutions where this might seem to be clearly the case, it is important that the availability of basic rights should not be further reduced by the requirements of a behaviour modification programme.

49.   In the evidence submitted to the Working Party, a considerable body of opinion took the view that a basic standard of care should be available as of right; the use of reinforcement techniques in therapeutic programmes should involve exclusively the provision of goods or privileges which improve on this basic standard.

50.   While this evidence suggested that reinforcement techniques should always be positive, it was represented to us that, in certain cases, it might be necessary to restrict access to any or all of the material goods, activities or events which can serve as reinforcements contingent upon the performance of a particular pattern of desired behaviour. In these circumstances, general concern was expressed that such deprivation should be strictly temporary and that basic standards of care should be appropriately safeguarded. Moreover, it is the view of the Working Party that, where behaviour modification programmes involve restricted availability of goods or privileges, they should invariably be subject to the patients' consent. (See Chapter 3, paragraph 31).

Aversion Treatment

51.   In technical terminology an aversive stimulus is one whose *removal* as the result of an appropriate response leads to the strengthening of that response. For example, an animal may learn to avoid an electric shock by pressing a lever which prevents delivery of shock. This is known as *avoidance conditioning* and some use of it has been made in behaviour therapy, eg in the treatment of

enuresis. The term *aversion treatment,* however is more generally used for procedures in which an unpleasant or even mildly painful stimulus (eg weak electric shock) is applied with a view to weakening, and perhaps abolishing altogether, a form of behaviour which is considered to be actually or potentially harmful to the patient himself or to other persons.

52. Aversion treatment involves what is technically known as *negative reinforcement* and is explained in Appendix I. While it, too, has found limited application in behaviour therapy (eg in the treatment of chronic alcoholism), it seldom plays any part in behaviour modification programmes using groups or larger units.

53. At the same time, group behaviour modification programmes not infrequently involve a procedure known as *time-out* (See Appendix I for definition), in which positive reinforcement (reward) is temporarily withheld. In clinical practice, this is often achieved by isolating the patient for a brief period from his ordinary social setting. Time-out from positive reinforcement is often equated with mild punishment and may therefore be said to constitute an aversive form of treatment.

54. Any form of aversion treatment, however mild, evidently creates an ethical dilemma. The Working Party gave much thought to this dilemma and came to the conclusion that mild forms of deprivation, in particular time-out, can be regarded as acceptable provided that they are used sparingly and in the context of a behaviour modification programme in which the major emphasis is placed upon positive reinforcement. On the other hand, the Working Party considered that techniques which may cause appreciable discomfort or even mild degrees of pain should be employed only as a last resort when all forms of behaviour modification based on positive reinforcement have been tried and have failed. In such cases, it was thought advisable that aversion treatment should be used only after full interdisciplinary discussion and subject to the usual consent procedures, which should preferably be in writing (See para 31).

Chapter 5
RESPONSIBILITY

55. The issue of responsibility in the implementation of behaviour modification programmes greatly exercised the Working Party throughout its deliberations and obtruded itself constantly in discussion of the issues considered in the earlier chapters of this Report. Apart from its sole legally qualified member (Mr M Edwardes-Evans), no member of the Working Party possessed a concept of responsibility going appreciably beyond that accepted, implicitly at least, in the practice of his or her own profession or any special knowledge or experience of its legal implications. None the less, the Working Party was quick to recognise that the practice of behaviour modification should proceed in a manner which, while consistent with those conceptions of responsibility traditionally held in the professions from which its practitioners are drawn, should at the same time endeavour to adapt them to the essentially multidisciplinary (or "trans-professional") character of this form of therapeutic endeavour.

56. In order to specify guidelines which might help to achieve this aim, the Working Party was greatly assisted by an able analysis of the concept of legal responsibility prepared by Mr Edwardes-Evans and reproduced as Appendix IX. In it, he makes the point that the term "Responsible Medical Officer", defined as being the Medical Practitioner in charge of the treatment of a detained patient, is only applicable in the context of the relevant statute of the 1959 Mental Health Act and has no legal meaning outside the context of the Act. He further points out that a legal duty of care towards patients is owed by each separate individual who may be concerned with his treatment, the required standard of such treatment varying according to the skills and qualifications of the individual concerned. In the event of mishap, the Court is not concerned with "accountability" in the managerial sense provided that the consultant in charge has exercised proper care in delegating individual authority.

57. It would appear from this analysis that, in carrying through programmes of behaviour modification in institutions within the National Health Service, every member of the clinical (or multi-disciplinary) team exercises responsibility in accordance with his qualifications and professional training. It would likewise appear that the consultant has a duty to ascertain, in so far as is reasonably possible, that the qualifications and skills of those to whom he delegates authority in the conduct of behaviour modification programmes are of an acceptable standard. This matter is discussed further in Para 61.

Good Practice and Multi-Professional Teamwork

58. For all patients admitted to hospital, there will be an NHS consultant in overall charge of all aspects of treatment. Further, it is the consultant's duty to ensure so far as possible that the resources of the hospital are made available to provide the range of clinical services that his patient requires. When a patient is discharged from hospital or treated as an outpatient, the general practitioner and the consultant should agree between themselves the location of the medical responsibility. In the case of some chronic diseases, eg schizophrenia, it may be appropriate that this responsibility be shared.

59. In addition to receiving medical treatment all patients will receive some form of nursing care and treatment and some may require clinical services from other professional staff. It is increasingly the fact that non-medical professional staff possess knowledge and experience in diverse fields (eg nursing, psychology, remedial education) of which a medical consultant can have only limited and very general knowledge. It is thus often the case that non-medical staff are required to provide specific clinical services, responsibility for which rests with the individual to whom referral has been made. He is expected to act responsibly within the terms of his own training and professional experience. Essentially, every profession has its own competence and its members are responsible for decisions within their own sphere. This implies that members of each profession acknowledge the limits of their own competence.

60. The position of all professional trainees deserves special mention. A trainee is not absolved from responsibility but delegation of authority is

22

abused if a trainee is required to carry out without adequate supervision, a procedure for which he is insufficiently trained.

61. In his work with members of other professions within a hospital, the consultant is entitled to assume that the health authorities, in appointing a particular individual to a post, have satisfied themselves that such an individual has been adequately trained and possesses the necessary qualifications for satisfactory discharge of his duties at an appropriate level of expertise. In general, therefore, he may legitimately expect on the part of nonmedical professional staff, competence in such treatment or remedial methods as fall within the sphere of their professional training and experience. At the same time, in referring patients to non-medical staff in connection with a particular form of treatment (including remedial training), the consultant has still the duty to ensure that those to whom referral is made are capable of treating at a level and in a manner appropriate to the requirements of each particular patient under his care. It will be appreciated that the consultant-in-charge may delegate his responsibility but cannot abrogate it. In this connection, reference should be made to the Statement of Policy of the Royal College of Psychiatrists regarding the ultimate responsibility of the consultant in the National Health Service.*

62. In drawing up a treatment programme a consultant should call upon the skills of his non-medical professional colleagues, discussing with them the needs of his patient and looking to them to provide specialised elements of care for which they possess particular competence and for which, as has been said, they assume an appropriate degree of responsibility. Multi-professional teamwork makes possible the mechanism whereby treatment programmes can be discussed and agreed between the professional groups concerned.

63. This concept of the multi-disciplinary team has arisen as the result of the many and complex developments in clinical practice which have made it virtually impossible for any one profession to possess thorough competence in other than its own sphere. As the range of clinical knowledge has widened so have a variety of professional groups emerged, each with its own specialised knowledge and expertise. The single-handed virtuoso of the past has been virtually supplanted by the clinical team and in psychiatric treatment these teams are for the most part multi-disciplinary.

64. These considerations are of particular relevance to the design and implementation of behaviour modification programmes in so far as the latter typically relate to the activities of a very considerable number of staff from different professional groups and their participation may entail some changes in traditional professional roles. For example, nurses, psychologists, occupational therapists, who formerly had relatively narrow and specialised roles, nowadays have a wider, more active and more integrated part to play in therapeutic endeavour. At the same time, it is necessary that staff from these and other relevant professional groups should retain sufficient autonomy within the multi-disciplinary team to enable them to make such adjustments in the implementation of a behaviour modification programme as may be demanded from the standpoint of their own particular professional outlook and practice.

---

*The Responsibilities of Consultant Psychiatrists within the National Health Service (Bulletin of the Royal College of Psychiatrists, September 1977)

23

65. It is in this context that the Working Party have considered where responsibility resides for decisions relating to behaviour modification programmes. While of course accepting that the consultant has an overall duty of care in seeing that all goes well with his patient, it is the opinion of the Working Party that non-medical professional staff, eg clinical psychologists and nurses, have clear responsibility for their specific contributions to either the design or the implementation of a programme, or to both (cf. para 57). For example, in the case of mentally handicapped patients who present primarily management and educational problems, it would seem fitting that non-medical personnel might well undertake the immediate decision making where their experience, competence and day-to-day involvement with the patients indicate that it is appropriate for them to do so. A clear recognition of their assumption of responsibility would add to their interest and involvement in therapeutic activity.

NOTE: In response to the preliminary circulation to them of the Working Party's Report the three parent bodies made a number of comments in relation to this Chapter. Their comments are summarised below.

The Royal College of Psychiatrists considered that the following sentences should be added to this Chapter: "The consultant has the responsibility of allowing the patient to commence on a programme, to continue with it and to withdraw him. It is his continuing responsibility to satisfy himself that the treatment is in the patient's best interests and discontinue treatment if it is not".

The British Psychological Society argued that the concepts expressed fail to reflect the concept of multi-disciplinary teamwork as practised in a clinical setting. In particular, statements concerning NHS consultant psychiatrists being "in overall charge of all aspects of treatment" and "delegating authority" were felt to be incompatible with the evolving patterns of teamwork. The Society instanced the Trethowan Report as a contribution to an ongoing exchange which is currently being furthered in discussions on responsibility between the British Psychological Society and the Royal College of Psychiatrists. The Society felt that the concept of responsibility may well be substantially revised over the next few years.

The Royal College of Nursing considered that the nurse has a responsibility towards care and treatment which will develop, restore, or maintain the independence of the patient. In certain circumstances the nurse will initiate a treatment programme where the activities involved are within the competence of the nurse and consistent with training received. In those situations where treatment is initiated by other professions the nurse has a right and duty to express an opinion in respect of its effect on the patient and/or the implications for staff.

Chapter 6
REVIEW BODIES

66. In the evidence submitted to us, there is a strong body of opinion to the effect that behaviour modification is in no sense unique among current methods of psychiatric treatment in giving rise to ethical questions. One might,

for instance, cite psychosurgery and certain types of drug treatment. Our remit is, however, confined to ethical aspects of behaviour modification and, in particular, to any aspect of its practice as may have a wider or different significance from that attaching to other forms of medical treatment. The Working Party considered at length the question of whether behaviour modification raised special issues of ethical import which could not be covered by the general argument that the responsibility of care alone, which the vast majority of workers in the field of mental health practice with devotion, is necessarily sufficient to allay disquiet or to control potential abuse. The Working Party rejected the general argument and agreed (one member, Dr C P Seager,* dissenting) that there should be a formal framework within which the practice of behaviour modification should be open to scrutiny and review in so far as its ethical aspects are concerned.

67. In addition to the minority view within the Working Party, two of the parent bodies were unable to accept the suggestions made by the Working Party. The Working Party felt, nonetheless, that the issues involved merited discussion within this report and that, consequently, the arguments should be outlined as a basis for possible further consideration.

68. All are clear that the highest professional standards have to be maintained and the public safeguarded. While at the same time freedom to take advantage of therapeutically appropriate training and skills is not jeopardised. Informal and sympathetic discussion between those responsible for the design and conduct of behaviour modification programmes, coupled with full freedom of information resulting from their implementation, should form the basis upon which safeguards are built. At the same time, attitudes towards the ethical issues which such programmes are apt to raise will depend to a considerable degree upon what is considered ethically acceptable and this is of course liable to undergo change in course of time. In consequence, the Working Party doubted whether reliance on professional standards alone provides a basis of sufficient breadth to allay possible anxieties among staff, patients, relatives, helpers and the general public.

69. Experience in the United States (cf Appendices VII and VIII) has shown that, without appropriate safeguards, behaviour modification programmes have on occasion been utilised purely for convenience in administration of an institution. This has led to a series of constitutionally and statutorily induced safeguards against possible abuses. Often, however, the law envisages safeguards in terms of rigid obligations and prohibitions. The Working Party believes that a compromise should be sought between the extremes of unrestrained professional authority on the one hand and rigid legal controls on the other.

70. Our enquiries disclosed that throughout the country a variety of behaviour modification programmes have been instituted, have died away or are progressing with varying degrees of vigour. Few, however, appear to have been reviewed by any relevant body either at the outset or subsequently and for the most part little or no regard had been paid to the ethical implications of what was being done. Indeed surprise was expressed in some quarters at the

---

*Dr C P Seager's views are presented in a paper entitled "Review Bodies—An Alternative View" appended to this Report (Appendix VI)

suggestion that behaviour modification programmes might give rise to ethical issues of any kind. None the less, it would seem that disquiet has been felt at the lack of a code of ethics for behaviour modification. Suggestions which were made to us included a statutory body comparable to the Mental Health Review Tribunals, a form of Health Advisory Service on a national basis and a committee structure at Area Health Authority level.

71. Of the seventeen professional bodies and other organisations which provided us with written evidence (cf. Appendix III), all but one expressed a view as to the desirability or otherwise of instituting Review Bodies to consider proposed behaviour modification programmes and to review their progress and outcome. It is noteworthy that, of these seventeen bodies, ten considered a review procedure of some kind desirable in principle, whereas three were opposed to any such procedure, except in the case of a programme involving an important element of research, in which case it could be referred to an existing Ethical/Research Committee.

72. As already noted, the Working Party, with one member dissenting, agreed that there should be a formal framework for review and scrutiny of the practice of behaviour modification. It was felt that such a framework should not be so rigid and bureaucratic as to discourage initiative in developing novel behaviour modification techniques or to interfere with the treatment of an individual patient when he is clearly in a position to assess what is involved in the programme and has signified his willingness to participate. It should, however, serve to protect patients from the diminution of values and dignities which can in extreme cases extend to deprivation or limitation of basic human rights. It could also counterbalance the possible adverse effects of over-enthusiasm in devising new and controversial programmes or from abuse or misuse of existing behavioural procedures.

73. There already exists a structure of ethical committees throughout the country the object of which is to safeguard patients, healthy volunteers and the reputation of investigators and their institutions in matters relating to clinical research. The concern of these committees is limited to research and does not extend to issues of treatment or practice. The official recommendation of the Royal College of Physicians in 1973 was that, in medical institutions in which clinical research is carried out, all projects should be approved by a group of doctors "who should be experienced clinicians with a knowledge of clinical research investigation and in addition there should be a lay member". Such a lay member should not be drawn from a paramedical sphere and the Department of Health and Social Security urges consideration of a member of the appropriate Community Health Council (CHC). Nevertheless it seemed impractical to clothe the problem of approval and/or control of behaviour modification programmes in the mantle of research. The Working Party felt that existing ethical/research committees (which in some areas do not appear even to exist) are inappropriate for this task.

74. The Working Party doubted whether the present Health Service structure could accommodate such specialised and yet wide ranging functions as were envisaged. As has been said, the existing ethical/research committees are inappropriate in so far as they are too limited in function and membership; the medical balance would be too high to be appropriate for assessment of behaviour modification programmes. The CHC's, on the other hand, might

seem too widely spread (as regards both number and function) and rather more 'consumer-orientated' than might be thought appropriate in view of the somewhat specialised approach and balance of interests which would be necessary to appraise such programmes. The structure and membership of Mental Health Review Tribunals might form the nucleus for review bodies but as at present constituted they do not seem suitable to deal with the type of work envisaged since a considerable number of professions other than those now represented might have to be co-opted on to them. To require each hospital to set up its own review body would be cumbersome, especially when the burden of committees is already heavy and the incidence and type of behaviour modification programmes throughout the area so varied. Review by internal bodies could also lead to criticism on the basis of the maxim that justice must be seen to be done.

75.   Review arrangements need to be sufficiently broadly based to cover all the essential and practical elements comprising any behaviour modification programme. In particular, an opportunity should be provided to look at the goals of a programme as well as the steps being taken to attain them. The question must be asked whether such goals are in the best interests of the patient or group of patients involved or merely directed towards getting jobs done in the hospital with minimal benefit to those undertaking them. There would need also to be scrutiny of the methods which are being used and an evaluation of the relative success or effectiveness of the programme when it had been completed. The aim in all cases would be to achieve and maintain standards which conformed to an acceptable national code of ethics.

76.   It is important to appreciate that a system of review cannot be confined to a proposed behaviour modification programme in isolation from its social setting. It must consider the effect of the programme not only on the patient but also on his relatives, and indeed on all those who may be associated, directly or indirectly, with its implementation, in all of whom a degree of anxiety may be aroused. Particular difficulties may arise in the provision of safeguards for the patients, particularly those so handicapped as to be considered incapable of giving initial consent or of understanding the methods to be employed, or where there is any doubt as to the validity of the consent given or obtained.

77.   In the light of these considerations the Working Party suggested that Behaviour Modification Review Committees be established throughout the country, initially at Regional Health Authority level. Their remit would be to cover all relevant activities in the Region whether in the Hospital or in the community, including those concerned with out-patients. Relevant activities would be all group or ward regimes in which the patients' privileges, money, goods and facilities are or may be manipulated in the interest of the behaviour modification programme, but not ordinarily individual programmes or programmes in institutions outside the area of responsibility of the DHSS. The Committees would act in an advisory capacity to institutions undertaking programmes of behaviour modification under the aegis of the National Health Service. The aim would be to assist development of programmes as opposed to retarding or inhibiting enterprise or innovation in the development of new or untried behaviour modification procedures.

78.   As envisaged by the Working Party the Review Committee would have lay and professional members, including those with appropriate professional

background and expertise in behaviour modification and those with knowledge of the law, more especially in relation to the rights of individuals. The Review Committee would be empowered to meet in public and required to do so when programmes rather than individuals were being discussed.

79. The remit of the Review Committee would be to appraise, monitor and if necessary comment upon all ethical aspects of behaviour modification within their region. In addition, they could where necessary constitute an independent panel to which matters relating to behaviour modification in which patients are incapable of giving consent or where relatives are unavailable could be referred (See Paragraph 36). The Working Party suggested that Review Committees might also receive and hear relevant complaints.

80. The Review Committee would be empowered to call for details of and to examine at will or on request all or any programmes of behaviour modification within the Region; to visit any hospitals or other places in which behaviour modification may be or is being practised; to interview all relevant medical and other associated staff, patients or relatives or others concerned in any way in any behaviour modification programme. Details of all programmes of behaviour modification planned or operating in the Region would have to be notified to the Review Committee as soon as practicable, within the framework as outlined in paragraph 72. The Review Committee would also be notified of all programmes which had been completed or terminated, with reasons. The ethical content of all programmes of behaviour modification in operation in any given Region should be reviewed annually.

81. As already noted, one member of the Working Party dissented from the proposal for Review Committees. Dr C P Seager saw Review Committees as stifling initiatives for treatment because of bureaucratic requirements and that this effect would be particularly damaging to novel and less well established treatments. There would be difficulties in staffing the Committees in general and in particular with individuals with expertise. The concept of Review Committees could spread to other forms of treatment and therefore interfere with progress in other fields. Improvements in complaints procedures were already being considered.

82. The Royal College of Nursing saw the suggestion for Review Committees as an area for further discussion. They expressed the general feeling that there is a need for some form of monitoring system.

83. The Royal College of Psychiatrists opposed the concept of Review Committees on the grounds that they could not fulfil their purpose as advisory panels and that therefore legislation would be needed to give them statutory powers. Such powers would encroach on professional clinical freedoms and would as such be alien to the principle and spirit of the Health Service. The College saw the responsibility for monitoring programmes resting with the Consultant-in-Charge and felt that behaviour modification was, as all treatments or services, controlled by professional and ethical standards and recognised complaints procedures. The College considered that there might be a body similar to the Mental Welfare Commission (for Scotland).

84. The British Psychological Society was unconvinced of the need for Review Committees and held that existing safeguards should be strengthened rather than new structures created. Existing complaints procedures should be

made more effective and greater reliance should be placed on the role of the professions in ensuring standards of professional conduct with "multidisciplinary teamwork" ensuring informed decision making. The Society suggest, however, that if Committees to review treatment programmes were to be required, they should not be set up at Regional level since these would be too cumbersome in operation and remote from clinical practice. Instead, they should be based on existing Research Ethics Committees which operate increasingly at Sector or District level. The Society were also concerned that, should Committees be established, they should be involved with all aspects of care of long-stay and mental handicapped persons and in particular with those aspects of treatment involving aversive stimuli (including the use of time-out rooms) or actual or potential restriction of patients' rights and privileges, regardless of the label given to the programme. In addition the Review Committee might investigate any programme about which there had been a formal complaint. Clinicians should be encouraged to refer any programme which may raise ethical issues or be misconstrued by patients, colleagues or the lay public. The Society noted that the Working Party did not specify the duties or rights of the Review Committees in the event of their not being satisfied with a programme which is proposed or in existence. The Society suggests that, should advice and persuasion fail to bring essential changes, the Review Committee should not have executive powers but rather powers of reference to relevant professional managers or senior colleagues of the clinician and to the relevant employing authority and appropriate body.

85.   In the light of the objections summarised in paras 81, 83 and 84, the Working Party resolved to withdraw its original recommendation that Behaviour Modification Review Committees be established. It nevertheless expresses the hope that the advantages or otherwise of establishing review arrangements for programmes of behaviour modification will continue to be widely debated.

Chapter 7
TRAINING

86.   The main professions concerned with the planning and implementation of behaviour modification programmes are psychiatry, clinical psychology and nursing of the mentally ill and mentally handicapped. While individual members of all three professions have acquired proficiency in the conduct of behaviour modification methods of treatment, there has until recently, been no attempt on the part of any of the three professional groups involved to establish minimum standards of competence. In consequence, behaviour modification programmes have on occasion been started by staff who are inadequately qualified.

87.   In addition to those three main groups, our questionnaire returns (See Paragraphs 10 and 11, and Appendix II) indicate that members of several other professional groups might on occasion be concerned in the operation of behaviour modification programmes. These include Occupational Therapists (the next most common profession involved), Social Workers, Physiotherapists, Speech Therapists, Art Therapists and Teachers. The

qualifying training in none of these professions requires practical experience in behaviour modification though, in several, the theoretical basis of the methods in use is covered to a certain extent.

88. Many schemes of behaviour modification have been started by the enthusiasm of nursing staff and others with a high degree of day-to-day patient contact. A number of these have failed through lack of overall planning and insufficient preparation of others, both inside and outside the institution, who have not understood what the treatment programme involved. The evidence derived from our Questionnaire Survey (cf Appendix II) further shows that both psychiatrists and psychologists have initiated behaviour treatment programmes with little or no prior training or practical experience and nor have the nurses running the programmes.

Existing Qualifying Training and Post-Basic Training Courses

(i) *Nurses*

89. Statutory training for nurses in the fields of mental handicap and mental illness is controlled by the Statutory Nursing Bodies within the United Kingdom. In the relevant syllabuses, those for parts of the Register of Mental Nurses (RMN) and Nurses for the Mentally Subnormal (RNMS and RNMD), there is a clear emphasis upon the nurse's function in training, management and education of patients. In both the mental illness and mental handicap fields, there is a disparity between the formal syllabus and its interpretation in the practical training situation. The shortage of trained Nurse Teachers is acute throughout the National Health Service and is especially acute in the Mental Handicap Training Schools.

90. Opportunities for post-qualification training for nurses in all areas have recently improved markedly as a result of the setting up of the Joint Board of Clinical Nursing Studies. Courses in "Behaviour Modification for the Mentally Handicapped" and in "Adult Behavioural Psychotherapy" have been introduced, are now running and are to be welcomed, although the total output of these courses is at present extremely small. In Scotland, the Committee of Clinical Nursing Studies has introduced a syllabus on "Behaviour Therapy in Psychiatric and Mental Handicap Nursing".

(ii) *Psychiatrists*

91. With the present-day emphasis on instruction in Behavioural Science in pre-medical education, there is an increasing probability that basic behavioural concepts will be included in the preclinical education of medical students. A few may also receive some practical experience of behaviour modification in the course of their clinical training, though this will obviously vary from one medical school to another. Numbers may be expected to grow if more behaviourally orientated psychiatrists are appointed to the staff of University Departments of Psychiatry.

92. Post-basic training in psychiatry is now principally directed at the Membership examination of the Royal College of Psychiatrists, although a number of University and Medical teaching bodies still offer the Diploma in Psychological Medicine (DPM). Until a trainee psychiatrist has obtained either a DPM or the Preliminary Test of the MRC Psych, no assumptions can be

made with regard to his knowledge of behaviour modification. Following the first Report of the Joint Committee on Higher Psychiatric Training, the requirement has been laid down that all specialist psychotherapists should have knowledge and supervised experience in behavioural therapies and be familiar with their use both in individual and in small and large group settings.

(iii) *Clinical Psychologists*

93.   It may be assumed that all graduates from British Universities who have obtained Honours Degrees in which Psychology was taken as a main subject will have received formal instruction in behaviour theory and many will also have received some instruction in behavioural methods of treatment. Such persons are qualified to enter the National Health Service as Probationer Clinical Psychologists.

94.   Post-graduate professional training in clinical psychology leads to a higher University Degree (as a rule, the MSc) or to the Diploma in Clinical Psychology of the British Psychological Society. Clinical psychologists will ordinarily have received some supervised experience in behaviour therapy in individual cases and many will also have had experience of group and ward applications of behavioural methods.

(iv) *Inter-Disciplinary Training Courses*

95.   Short training courses (often called 'Workshops') have been organised by a very small number of Health Services and professional organisations. These tend to be sporadic and are usually of only 2-5 days duration, but some offer a good mixture of theoretical instruction and practical training. Such courses have been innovative and stimulating and have introduced many people to basic ideas in behaviour therapy.

96.   Unfortunately, our Questionnaire returns (cf Appendix II) indicate that some senior hospital staff may have mistakenly taken attendance at such a 'Workshop' to constitute in itself an adequate training in behaviour courses, underlining the need for longer training under on-going supervision. They do, however, have a special value when used as on-site training to prepare administrators, nursing officers and other staff of a particular hosptial for a specific new behaviour modification programme.

Recommendations

97.   The Working Party have considered carefully priorities in training. Whereas the evidence received by the Working Party placed emphasis primarily on training needs in the individual professions from which workers in behaviour modification are drawn, it was felt that, in the first instance at least, training resources should be concentrated on establishing a body of psychiatrists, psychologists and nurses with substantial theoretical knowledge and practical experience in behaviour modification. This body would provide a nucleus for the development, as and where appropriate, of more formal training arrangements, which might be either interdisciplinary or adapted more specifically to the needs of particular professional groups whose members were likely to become active in behaviour modification.

31

98. Although everyone involved in behaviour modification programmes brings to it his own unique background and outlook, the essentially collaborative nature of most behavioural programmes means that training should have a multi-disciplinary character. Professional boundaries may have to be crossed and training in managing and supervising members of other professions may become essential.

99. Insofar as introducing training is concerned, the Working Party recommend that a scheme of 'Workshops' and in-service training be instituted, giving guidelines on the type of teaching experience required in different treatment settings. Specialised post-qualifying training will be needed for those staff taking responsibility for the development of programmes, and this is seen as a particularly high priority.

100. Training in any method of treatment is not completed by attending the last lecture or practical of a course and some method of continuing evaluation of performance is essential. Courses should be assessed from the point of view of the degree to which they inculcate practical skill rather than formal knowledge.

101. It is most desirable that staff who have had a certain, if limited, amount of specialised training should receive a continuing degree of supervision and have opportunities for consultation with more experienced colleagues. This is particularly important for direct-care treatment staff, who may otherwise become rigid or even grossly incorrect in their application of behavioural procedures.

102. In the case of many programmes, adequate preparation or training of persons other than the professional staff of the institutions is essential. Hospital ancillary staff, patients' relatives, and referral and follow-up agencies in the community may all require information and guidance if a programme affects their area of activity. In training, therefore, the importance of establishing and maintaining all such contacts should be stressed, thereby incorporating into the treatment programme all those likely to be involved with the patient, in particular his relatives and visitors. Training schemes should give special attention to the need to keep relatives and others closely concerned fully informed about programmes of behaviour modification and their progress.

103. Instructors generally should aim to develop an appreciation of the importance of clearly stated aims and of adequate systems of evaluating results.

104. Every encouragement should be given to research with a view to the refinement of existing techniques and the development of new ones.

Chapter 8
SUMMARY AND RECOMMENDATIONS

105. The Working Party wishes to make the following recommendations with a view to establishing guidelines for the practice of behaviour modification:—

1. Full information concerning the aims and methods of a behaviour modification programme should always be available to the patient and his relatives. Explanation to relatives is particularly important in cases in which the patient may be incapable of fully understanding the import of what is said to him or of giving valid consent to treatment.

2. Information in appropriate form about an actual or proposed behaviour modification programme should always be made available to the staff of the institution concerned, including those staff members not directly involved in its implementation. Cases may however arise, particularly in individual behaviour therapy, in which it may be thought undesirable to discuss a behaviour modification programme specifically designed for a particular patient with staff other than those directly concerned with its design and conduct unless the patient first gives his consent.

3. Consent to participate in a behaviour modification programme should always be obtained from the patient, or, where he or she is incapable of giving valid consent, agreement from the nearest relatives should be sought. In circumstances in which relatives are unavailable, agreement might be sought from a 'third party advocate' or an independent panel.

4. In general, oral consent to treatment is thought sufficient. If, however, the programme involves re-scheduling of access to food or money, appreciably limiting visits or the quantity of leave, necessitates brief periods of isolation or physical restraint, or employs procedures which might on occasion cause a degree of discomfort, the person in charge of the programme may consider that written consent should be obtained. The intention would be to avoid any subsequent dispute as to what has been agreed.

5. All patients in National Health Service institutions have the right to expect a high standard of professional care, acceptable standards of accommodation and subsistence, and the right to retain their own goods and money subject to certain statutory regulations. These rights and privileges must be meticulously respected by all who design or implement programmes of behaviour modification.

6. Where a behaviour modification programme implies a measure of restriction of access to a patient for which consent has been forthcoming, the reasons for it should be carefully explained to his or her relatives or other visitors and their cooperation sought. Restrictions on access, which should be minimal, should under no circumstances exceed two weeks.

7. Where a programme implies restricting availability of goods or privileges as an essential feature of its design, such restriction should be strictly temporary and subject to appropriate consent, monitoring and supervision. It is essential to ensure in all cases that basic standards of care are appropriately safeguarded.

8. It is accepted by the Working Party that the use of aversion treatment in behaviour modification poses an ethical dilemma. Although seeing no complete solution, the Working Party recommend that mild deprivation procedures, eg time-out, are as a rule acceptable, provided that they are used sparingly in the context of a behaviour modification programme based for the most part on positive reinforcement, ie 'reward'. On the other hand, it is strongly recommended that techniques which may cause discomfort or even

mild degrees of pain (eg weak electric shock) should be employed only as a last resort when techniques making use of positive reinforcement have been tried and have failed. Aversion treatment should in any case be used only after full inter-disciplinary discussion and subject to the usual consent procedures, which should preferably be in writing.

9. The practice of behaviour modification is made possible largely by acceptance of the multi-disciplinary therapeutic team. This concept has wide application in contemporary medicine, not least in psychiatry. We see no reason why an appropriate measure of authority should not be delegated to non-medical personnel active in the practice of behaviour modification in National Health Service institutions, provided that the patient's consultant is satisfied that such personnel are competent to discharge the requisite degree of responsibility. Within such a team, responsibility is governed by the general principle that every member of it is legally responsible for his own behaviour and must act appropriately within the limits imposed by his professional status, knowledge and experience. The Working Party accepts this principle. At the same time, it wishes to draw to the attention of the Department of Health and Social Security the fact that considerable debate regarding issues of responsibility in the implementation of behaviour modification programmes will continue to exist.

10. In order to safeguard the interests of both patients and professional staff, as well as to allay anxiety in the community generally, the Working Party initially recommended, with one member dissenting, that the Department of Health and Social Security be advised to establish Behaviour Modification Review Committees at Regional Authority level. Their remit would be to scrutinise all programmes of behaviour modification within the Region, to monitor their progress and assess their outcome. But in view of the substantial objections to this proposal advanced by two of the three parent bodies, it was agreed that this recommendation be withdrawn. Nonetheless, the Working Party expresses the hope that the desirability or otherwise of establishing formal review arrangements for programmes of behaviour modification will continue to be widely debated.

11. The Working Party has made a number of general recommendations relating to training in the practice of behaviour modification (Paragraphs 97-104). It is recommended that, in order to establish the necessary guidelines for training, the first step should be to build up the number of psychiatrists, psychologists and nurses with substantial knowledge and practical experience in behaviour modification, who could offer appropriate advice and guidance to members of their own professions and to others.

12. The Working Party recommends the further development of in-service training schemes and inter-disciplinary 'Workshops' in order to promote wider understanding and active use of behavioural methods and their application. Also recommended is the establishment of specialised further training posts for staff likely to take responsibility for the development and conduct of behavioural modification programmes. The multi-disciplinary character of behaviour modification means that some professional boundaries will be crossed and some professional roles re-defined. Courses of instruction should take account of these consequences.

13. The Working Party recommend that all those involved in instruction in behaviour modification should aim to foster an appreciation of the need for clearly stated aims and procedures and of adequate methods for evaluating results.

14. Every encouragement should be given to research in the field of behaviour modification.

The Working Party would like most sincerely to thank Mr F J Lewis and Miss J A Vass of the Department of Health and Social Security for their invaluable administrative and secretarial help.

Appendix I
BEHAVIOUR MODIFICATION

1.   The term *behaviour modification* has been widely used in recent years, though not always consistently and its connotations have not been without a degree of ambiguity. It is therefore important to consider how the current usage of the term has evolved and to identify the sense in which it has been understood by the Working Party.

2.   The earliest systematic usage of the term was by a group of clinical psychologists in the United States. They adopted it to express a particular viewpoint towards abnormal behaviour and to distinguish this viewpoint from that prevailing in contemporary psychological medicine. They sought to avoid explanation in terms either of "medical models" (ie abnormal behaviour considered as the outcome of illness or dysfunction) or in terms of assumed mental processes that could not be observed directly (eg abnormal feelings or beliefs) and to restrict themselves to descriptive accounts of *observable* behaviour and of the environmental circumstances in which it took place. Their object was thus to establish functional relationships between the environment and behaviour, an approach which owes its origin to Amercian behaviourist psychology and which today is particularly associated with the work and outlook of B F Skinner.

3.   The term *behaviour modification* has therefore come to mean a systematic approach to the understanding and treatment of abnormal behaviour, emphasising its environmental determinants rather than its possible origins in mental or physical illness. Its aim is systematically to manipulate events or occurrences in a patient's environment with a view to achieving a specific therapeutic target or goal. This goal is always specified in terms of *desired behaviour* rather than of improvement or cure in a conventional medical sense.

4.   Within this approach to clinical problems, a number of techniques have been introduced, based on experiments with both animal and human subjects, the results of which have led to a body of principles referred to collectively as *behaviour theory*. Many of these techniques make use of what is termed *operant conditioning,* which has found wide application in clinical practice. While it is neither necessary (nor indeed possible) to describe these techniques in detail here, they almost all make use of what is called *reinforcement*, which is as a rule positive and can be roughly equated with *reward*. More technically, a *reinforcer* is defined as any event which either increases or maintains the frequency of occurrence of a particular pattern of behaviour upon which it has been made dependent. It is a purely empirical matter to determine whether, and in what circumstances, a particular event is a reinforcer. The concept of reinforcement serves to direct attention to the important influence which some environmental events may come to exert over behaviour to which they are related but it does not ascribe this influence to any assumed inherent qualities of those events, eg that they are pleasant or fulfil an expectation. If a reinforcer in this empirical sense, can be identified and related appropriately to a desirable pattern of behaviour, it will increase the frequency with which such behaviour is displayed.

5.   Changes may be achieved by a progressive procedure in which the reinforcer is gradually made dependent on successive approximations to the final target behaviour which it is hoped to establish. This is known as *shaping*. Once a desired pattern of behaviour has been established, it may be maintained in the behavioural repertoire by continuing to make reinforcers dependent upon it, though not necessarily on every occasion on which that behaviour occurs (*intermittent reinforcement*). Behaviour may be channelled into appropriate contexts by a gradual process ("fading") which differentiates those situations in which a specified pattern of behaviour will be followed by reinforcement from those in which it will not (*discriminative control*). Thus a specific technology has emerged for constructing and maintaining what are thought to be appropriate or desirable behavioural repertoires in patients, it being suggested that abnormal behaviour may, to some extent at least, be an accidental result of unprogrammed relationships between that behaviour and reinforcers in an unplanned environment.

6.   Allied to this essentially constructive approach, procedures are sometimes introduced which are specifically designed to *decrease* the frequency with which *undesirable* patterns of behaviour occur. Thus, a pattern of behaviour may be maintained by uncontrolled relationships with reinforcers and its frequency of occurrence may therefore be decreased by ensuring that it is no longer followed by a reinforcer (*extinction*). It may also be possible to specify environmental events which serve to *decrease* the frequency of behaviours on which they have been made dependent. Such events, so-called *punishers,* are specified purely in terms of their effects on behaviour in particular situations, and inherent qualities, such as that they are painful or disliked by the subject, are not ascribed to them.

7.   Since the initial development of the behaviour modification approach, the phrase has come to be used by others of less well-defined theoretical persuasions. As a result, more emphasis has come to be placed on *techniques* of behaviour modification, and some would choose to *define* behaviour modification wholly in terms of techniques. Unfortunately, the criteria for determining which techniques are truly based on established principles of behaviour theory and which are not have become somewhat uncertain. There is, for example, a tendency for *any* effective technique which changes behaviour or achieves an improvement in it, even if this is poorly specified, to be termed behaviour modification. Although this wide and imprecise usage of the term is not without its dangers, it has at least served to alert the public and professional workers of different disciplines (psychiatrists, nurses, teachers etc) to the environmental control that is, or may be, exerted in institutions, not always in contexts which would be readily agreed to be therapeutic.

8.   It is, of course, a futile exercise to try to insist that a particular connotation of a phrase is its "proper" meaning and the Working Party has made no attempt to do this. It has recognised that behaviour modification has become an imprecise term, yet it has also to be borne in mind that it has come to refer to a general area of public and professional concern, as is emphasised by the recommendations in the Report on certain events at Napsbury Hospital which can be described as involving behaviour modification only in a very broad and ill-defined way. The Working Party therefore itself attempted to proceed with a definition according to which *behaviour modification* comprehends both behaviour therapy with individual patients or small groups

and projects working within large groups such as wards or units within hospitals. In either case, however, it assumed that the procedures involved were based, more or less directly, on the general principles outlined in this Appendix. In view of its *raison d'etre,* the Working Party has concentrated especially on projects of the latter type, in which token-economy and related techniques find major application.

9.   The broad definition of *behaviour modification* adopted by the Working Party entailed that any of the re-educational methods based upon principles of learning theory should be classed as methods of behaviour modification, even if some were based on principles which depart in certain respects from those governing operant conditioning as defined by Skinner and others and summarised above. Among the methods which the Working Party considered appropriate to include in its review of behaviour modification are positive reinforcement, time-out, aversive treatment, token economy and desensitisation (see *Note* for definition of these terms). The Working Party intended that its more constrained definition of behaviour modification would none the less be sufficiently broad as to be of relevance to other procedures not universally regarded as programmes of behaviour modification, at all events in so far as ethical issues are concerned.

Notes

The following (relatively technical) definitions of some terms commonly used in connection with behaviour modification are appended:

(i) *Operant conditioning:* operant conditioning is a procedure in which the consequences of a specified pattern of behaviour are manipulated with a view to changing the frequency of that behaviour. Consequences which increase the frequency of behaviour are defined as positive reinforcers.

(ii) *Positive reinforcement:* The process of increasing the frequency of a specified pattern of behaviour by making the delivery of a selected environmental event dependent upon its occurrence.

(iii) *Negative reinforcement:* the process of increasing the frequency of a pattern of behaviour by making the removal or avoidance of a selected environmental event dependent on the behaviour in question.

(iv) *Time-out* (from positive reinforcement): the temporary removal of established opportunities for positive reinforcement. This is often achieved in clinical practice by physically removing the patient from his normal social settings and placing him in a barren room for a short period. Time-out from positive reinforcement has been shown to act as a "punisher" in the learning laboratory, ie, in many experiments it has led to a decrease in the frequency of the pattern of behaviour on which it is made dependent.

(v) *Aversion treatment:* this was interpreted to mean any treatment which includes the delivery of an aversive event. In technical terminology, an aversive stimulus is one whose *removal* as the result of the occurrence of a specified pattern of behaviour leads to an *increase* in the frequency of that behaviour. However, the Working Party also had in mind here procedures which include painful or unpleasant events, including those in which such events are *delivered* dependent upon behaviour in the hope of *decreasing* its frequency of occurrence.

(vi) *Token-economy:* a system which is often applied to all the individuals in a social unit such as a ward, and which has been described by some as a motivational system. Positive reinforcement (see above) has its greatest effect on the frequency of the patterns of behaviour which immediately precede the reinforcer. In token economies, a tangible signal (token) is given to a patient immediately after he produces an appropriate pattern of behaviour. The tokens are retained by the patient, and may ultimately be exchanged for what he chooses as goods or luxuries additional to those given in the ordinary course of events. If a token used in this way proves to increase the frequency of the behaviour which it follows, it is said to be a *conditioned reinforcer,* ie, one which has acquired its influence over behaviour as a result of the conditions in which it is used.

(vii) *Desensitisation:* a group of procedures for decreasing patients' emotional reactions to specific situations or objects, reactions which lead to maladaptive behaviour designed to avoid such situations or objects. The essence of these procedures is that the patient is exposed to a controlled sequence of situations or objects which increasingly resemble those giving rise to the dysfunction. Desensitisation is often used in conjunction with other procedures (including psychotherapy), and is sometimes interpreted as an example of the Pavlovian model of learning rather than as operant conditioning.

Appendix II
CURRENT BRITISH PRACTICE IN BEHAVIOUR MODIFICATION

At the beginning of the Working Party there was little clear information on the extent of behaviour modification practice in the United Kingdom apart from 3 short surveys published in 1972 and 1973. Accordingly every hospital in the country known to have psychiatric beds was contacted in May 1974 and asked whether any behaviour modification procedures were being carried out in the hospital. The 115 hospitals which responded in the affirmative to this first enquiry were contacted again in August and September 1974 and asked to provide information on 6 aspects of the behavioural treatment programmes in each hospital. These aspects were:
1. Type of programme or treatment.
2. Number of patients involved in each type of programme.
3. Type of patients involved.
4. The number and designation of staff assigned to each programme.
5. Details of staff training in behavioural methods.
6. Contacts with non-professional, voluntary, or community workers.

Since there was no standard reply form, completed answers did not all follow this outline, so the answers from different hospitals are not strictly comparable. Nor did they always reflect accurately the total picture of activity in a hospital, according to the first-hand knowledge of some members of the Working Party.

However, a number of general conclusions can be made from the survey. Table 1 shows the distribution of responses among different counties and different categories of hospital. It is noteworthy that the proportion of mental handicap hospitals providing details of programmes is higher than the proportion of mental illness hospitals.

Programmes in teaching or general hospitals with mental illness beds

The great majority of behavioural work going on was individual behaviour therapy, with up to 28 patients in treatment at any one time. The type of patient seen was principally neurotic out-patients, with obsessional-compulsive and phobic conditions the most frequently mentioned specific problems. Small-group treatment on a behavioural basis was going on in two hospitals. Because of this emphasis on acute work the staff most commonly involved in treatment were psychologists and psychiatrists, with little mention made of other staff apart from nurses.

Programmes in hospitals for the mentally ill

Over half the hospitals mentioned the use of individual behaviour therapy with neurotic patients, with one hospital reporting 200 patients in treatment at a time. Several comments were made about the prevalence of middle-aged women, and reference was made to the treatment of sexual problems in addition to phobic and obsessional problems. Token economy programmes were reported in two-fifths of the hospitals, the great majority of these programmes being for chronic psychiatric patients. The token programme varied in size from seven to 45 patients.

A quarter of the hospitals mentioned specific group programmes of various types, dealing with chronic patients, teaching social skills, reducing phobic and obsessional problems, and treating children. The size of the groups ranged from small groups of two or three to larger groups of 30, though the larger group sizes represented the total number of patients in treatment, and were

Table 1

	England	Scotland	Wales	N. Ireland	Replied no information	No reply	Total
Teaching/General Hospital with Mental Illness beds	13	—	—	—	2	1	16
Mental Illness Hospitals	32	7	2	2	3	8	54
Mental Handicap Hospitals	25	4	1	—	1	9	40
Special Hospitals	2	1	—	—	—	2	5
Total	72	12	3	2	6	20	115

Return rate: total replies received 82 pc
usable replies 77 pc

usually divided into smaller groups of unspecified size for treatment sessions. Ward-based individual programmes were mentioned in a few hospitals, most of these being for children with behaviour disorders or language disturbance.

In contrast to the Teaching/General Hospitals, psychiatrists were relatively less involved in these programmes, being mentioned specifically only half as frequently as psychologists. A number of occupational therapists and aides were involved, as well as a few teachers and social workers.

Although staffing ratios were requested for all hospital programmes, in most programmes it was not possible to arrive at any meaningful comparisons. However, it was possible to make a meaningful estimate in the case of token economy programmes, where the ratio of staff on duty at any one time to patients varied between 1:4 and 1:12, with a mean of 1:8.

Programmes in hospitals for the mentally handicapped

Token economies were mentioned in two-fifths of the hospitals, for groups ranging between four and 80 patients. The programmes were equally divided between those catering for the subnormal, and for the severely subnormal. An equal number of hospitals ran general ward or group programmes without tokens, for groups of mostly severely subnormal patients ranging in size between 3 and 20. Again a similar number of hospitals ran self-help skills programmes for predominantly severely subnormal patients (a third were children), with the total number of patients being treated varying from two to 45 per hospital.

A wide range of individual or specific programmes were mentioned by half the hospitals, treating such problems as incontinence and speech disability. Up to 100 patients in a hospital were being treated this way, some in groups of up to 21. About half the patients involved were severely subnormal, and about one-third for children or younger patients.

A notable feature of the mental handicap hospitals answers was a number of hospitals where a number of different types of programmes—up to seven—were operating at a time, involving a wide range of staff. Again the psychiatrists were mentioned less frequently than psychologists or nurses, but a wide range of staff, a number classed as Nursing Assistants, or "Therapists" were involved.

Programmes in the Special Hospitals

In one hospital a shortage of psychologists was specifically mentioned as the reason for the absence of behaviour modification programmes. In the other two a small number of patients are seen for individual or small group programmes, the types of problem being treated including lack of social skills, lack of self-help skills, illiteracy, and disruptive biting.

Staff training

One third of all hospitals gave some details of staff training. Half of these were described as "in-service training", "specific training as needed", etc. Less than one in fourteen of all hospitals indicated the existence of a clearly-thought out training scheme. It is worth noting that several hospitals mentioned "attendance at Conference (or Workshop)" as the sole evidence of training. Several also mentioned that training was carried out "at the beginning" or by "initial training course", with the implication that the same level of training was not necessarily available for new staff members.

Contacts with non-professional personnel

This question is of particular relevance to work with mentally handicapped and long-stay mentally-ill patients. Only a few hospitals gave any details of contact with relatives, volunteers, etc. However, a number stated that open visiting was in operation, or that relatives were involved as necessary. The replies to this question do not suggest anything restrictive or limiting about the programmes, only that relatives and volunteers are rarely involved systematically in treatment.

Appendix III
LIST OF PROFESSIONAL AND OTHER BODIES PROVIDING WRITTEN EVIDENCE

Association of Educational Psychologists
Association of University Teachers of Psychiatry
British Association for Behavioural Psychotherapy
British Association of Occupational Therapists
Campaign for the Mentally Handicapped
Department of Education and Science (Schools Branch)
Institute of Mental Subnormality
Institute of Psychiatry
Mental Patients' Union
Mind (National Association for Mental Health)
Northern Association for the Advancement of Behavioural Analysis and
    Change
Royal College of Nursing
The British Psychological Society
The British Society for the Study of Mental Subnormality
The Joint Board of Clinical Nursing Studies
The Patients Association
The Royal College of Psychiatrists

Questionnaire issued to Professional and other Bodies listed above

The following questions are designed to solicit your views on the desirable situation in relation to specific subjects deemed to be important in the implementation of programmes of behaviour modification:

1. Consent

When a patient is capable of giving consent, what procedure should be followed in obtaining consent?

When a patient is not capable of giving consent, what procedure should be followed:

  a. when a relative is available?
  b. when a relative is not available?
  c. when a relative is available but does not consent?

When a patient does not consent to treatment, under what conditions should treatment be given? (eg children, people who are detained patients under the MH Act).

Under what conditions should treatment be used as an emergency procedure without prior consent?

2. Responsibility

In the case of treatment carried out by (a) psychologists, (b) nurse therapists, (c) other groups, where should clinical responsibility lie?

Under what circumstances, if any, should they take overall clinical responsibility?

To what extent should the team nature of staffing of ward programmes alter responsibility?

3. Training

What should be the additional requirements for competence to carry out treatment in the case of (a) doctors, (b) psychologists, (c) nurses, (d) others?

Is the present training available adequate for work in behaviour modification as defined in the accompanying letter: if not, what changes are needed?

Should there be a formal evaluation of training and should those who have not demonstrated evidence of competence be precluded from responsibility?

4. Staffing

What are the relevant professional groups which ought to be involved in order to conduct a behaviour modification programme?

What staff-patient ratio in all grades of nursing staff is desirable?

What should be considered the minimum number of nurses in the ward at any one time for a given number of patients?

5. Access and information

Is there need for restriction of access (including visitors) to patients on group or individual programmes? If so, what people should have (a) restricted (b) unrestricted access?

To what extent should treatment and all treatment alternatives be fully explained to (a) the patient, (b) any other specified person?

What arrangements should be made for the dissemination of information and allowing opportunities for discussion?

6. *Control*

What should the basic rights of patients be in terms of availability of (a) food, (b) clothing, (c) accommodation, (d) goods, (e) cash, (f) professional care, (g) visitors?

Under what circumstances, if any, should manipulation of the above be incorporated in a treatment programme?

What degree of restriction of choice of goods or spending cash should be permitted in a programme?

7. *Review Bodies*

What should be the involvement, if any, of the local ethical and research committee?

Is there a need of initial and periodic review of schemes from local, Area or Regional level?

If review bodies were set up to monitor programmes what powers should they have and what should be the membership of the review body?

Appendix IV
LIST OF HOSPITALS VISITED BY MEMBERS OF THE WORKING PARTY

MENTAL ILLNESS HOSPITALS
Bexley Hospital, Bexley, Kent

Royal Edinburgh Hospital

Warlingham Park, Warlingham, Surrey

MENTAL HANDICAP HOSPITALS
Bryn-y-Neuadd Hospital, Llanfairfechan

Lea Hospital, Kidderminster

Northgate and District Hospital, Morpeth

Royal Earlswood Hospital, Redhill

Appendix V
LIST OF INDIVIDUALS INVITED TO GIVE ORAL OR WRITTEN EVIDENCE TO THE WORKING PARTY

Professor A Altschul
Professor of Nursing, Department of Nursing Studies, University of Edinburgh

Dr D H Clark
Consultant Psychiatrist, Fulbourn and United Hospitals, Cambridge

Mr C Gathercole
Principal Psychologist, Bryn-y-Neuadd Hospital, Llanfairfechan

Mr L O Gostin
"Justice"

Dr A Kushlick
Director of Health Care Evaluation Research Team, Wessex Regional Health
  Authority

Dr I M Marks
Consultant Psychiatrist, Bethlem Royal and Maudsley Hospitals
Chairman, British Association for Behavioural Psychotherapy

Professor T R Miles
Professor of Psychology, University College of Bangor

Dr A J Tierney
Lecturer in Nursing Studies, University of Edinburgh

Professor B A Williams, Provost of King's College, Cambridge; and formerly
Knightsbridge Professor of Philosophy, University of Cambridge

Appendix VI
REVIEW BODIES—AN ALTERNATIVE VIEW

C P Seager

"Ethics are injunctions to action and social action in particular given by a group or society to its members, by one individual to another and from an individual to himself—his conscience". Thus ethical guidelines may be a set of rules monitored by an inspectorate but are equally relevant if monitored by peers and probably more efficient if monitored by self. The problem therefore is to allow the spread of ethical values within the group so that each individual acts as his own inspector and failing this to allow adequate dissemination of information so that peer groups can arbitrate. Both of these techniques of monitoring are more efficacious than an external arbitrator since there is, apart from the sheer mechanics of control, an increased risk of mobilization of the esprit de corps of the unit under suspicion; there is thus the risk of denying information to the inspector. It is only where internal conditions are extremely poor and social cohesiveness breaks down that information is released to "Them" outside.

When considering the setting up of a supervisory organisation for any form of treatment or management within the National Health Service two important considerations must be recognised. First there is the fact that the vast majority of professional workers in the hospitals are engaged in activities which they believe are for the benefit of the people under their care. Inevitably there must be a very small minority who abuse their position for their own benefit but these are the exceptions. Problems more commonly occur where the

45

enthusiasm and concern get out of hand allowing errors of judgment concerning the means of achieving therapeutic ends.

Secondly it is important to ensure that any system of inspection, regulation and control places no interference with the treatment of patients particularly when they are in a position to assess the problems involved and give their willingness to participate. This question of consent and in particular the concept of "informed consent" is dealt with in the body of the Report. This warning about interference with the best interests of the patients' treatment must apply also to the question of the initiation of new and sometimes heretical methods of treatment which may be the product of individualistic thinking and yet may revolutionize the outcome of a particular condition. These problems are particularly difficult in psychiatry where treatments tend to be empirical rather than founded on laboratory based studies producing a rational treatment on the basis of biochemical, bacteriological or other findings.

It has been widely recognised that patients in hospital for a variety of reasons may be used for research purposes without understanding and giving valid consent to the procedures which are being used. Ethical Committees have been set up to monitor such research activities in order to ensure that the patient is protected from unreasonable and unknowing exploitation. Yet even these Ethical Committees operate as much from the pressures of public and peer group opinion as they do from a formal monitoring of the research procedure.

When one considers the question of treatment which is by definition aimed at alleviating the mental or physical "dis-ease" of the patient the situation is more complex. Where the individual is intelligent, mentally intact and wishes to enquire he can ensure he has the opportunity of understanding what is going to happen to him. It is interesting to note that many people do not take advantage of this ability, for a variety of reasons. Where the individual is incapacitated by virtue of intellectual disability or mental dysfunction the problem is inevitably more complicated and in the end he must rely on the good faith of those looking after him. The question under discussion is how best to ensure that those professional groups will indeed be concerned about the welfare of the individual and do their best to ensure his maximum benefit rather than allow considerations of personal convenience or the benefit of the institution to take precedence over that of the individual patient. This issue of the benefit of the individual in relation to the benefit of the community as a whole is not confined to psychiatric institutions and there have been many debates on problems of privacy, confidentiality, individual liberty and freedom in a variety of situations.

It is probably true to say that arising from these debates the single factor which stands out is the question of vigilance and a recognition that there are problems which have to be carefully considered.

In the issue before us it can be seen that the main problem is the pressure on relatives concerned for the patient to co-operate with any type of treatment which is seen to be of benefit to him though he himself may be unable to recognise this either because of disturbed thought process or intellectual incapacity. Pressures to guard against this paternalistic role of the caring professions have the disadvantage that the pendulum may swing too far and each individual would be expected to make judgment concerning matters over which he is in no position to assess the gains and losses. Indeed it raises the question of the value of expertise.

46

At present any control rests on the following factors:

1. Implicit faith in the caring professions.
2. Inter and intra disciplinary discussions concerning the merits of different types of treatments.
3. Propagation of information to the general public by the information media.
4. Complaints procedures both informal and formal.
5. Legal action against major transgressors.

Any or all of these processes can be strengthened in order to improve their capacity to monitor situations which may be considered potentially dangerous. There can be improvement in the selection and training of staff in order to enhance their capacity to look after patients properly. One finds that there is a vicious circle in that poor conditions lead to poor recruitment and this brings about worse conditions; public opinion must recognise the need for appropriate financial rewards and adequate working conditions in order to attract good quality staff.

The concept of multi-disciplinary therapeutic teams has already led to an improvement in the communication between the different professional groups involved. It is important that this process be speeded up by educational and professional advice in all the groups concerned.

Psychiatric institutions have for long been aware that there is need to keep the public informed of what goes on within their walls. It has taken many years to break down the isolation of the asylum behind high walls. Today there is more acceptance and less fear of mental illness and this is increasing with the introduction of psychiatric units in general hospitals. It is important to note that the fear and ignorance was not confined to the public at large but was also common in members of the medical and nursing profession who had no direct knowledge and experience of psychiatric problems. It is unfortunate that at the moment the greatest publicity arises from Committees of Enquiry looking into faults and disasters; it would be better if the publicity were shared more evenly so that the benefits and successes of treatment achieved equal prominence.

Where there is obstruction or rejection of legitimate enquiry there must be well publicized channels of complaint and access both on the part of patients and their relatives and also for staff who feel that there are procedures going on which are inappropriate or unethical. There must be facilities for private complaint outside the recognised formal management routes for those situations where an individual may feel that he would be victimised if he published his complaint. One must strike the right balance between lack of complaint because of fear of retribution and insidious backdoor anonymous complaints which undermine professional staff relationships.

Where there are serious infringements of the law, once legal proceedings are instituted the matter is of course outside the control of the professional staffs concerned.

One has to consider whether a Review Body is necessary and advisable to monitor formally the treatment procedures rather than encouraging informal monitoring on the lines already described. The objections to a Review Body may be summarized as follows:—

1. It will stifle initiative because of the bureaucratic requirements of submitting any proposal for treatment to such a Body. The further away

it is from the front line of hospital treatment the more hindrance there will be to active treatment.

2. Such monitoring will be particularly damaging to novel and less well established treatments.

3. The more specialised and unusual the treatment the less likely it will be to be assessed knowledgeably by non-specialists and yet the specialists will be fewer and more likely to be involved in the treatment procedure than a more widely accepted technique. This is probably particularly true of behaviour modification as it is now practised.

4. The concept of a Review Body for Behaviour Modification may be accepted as a precedent for all forms of treatment and will therefore interfere with progress in the wider field of psychiatry and of medicine in general.

5. It will add to the proliferation of committees already produced by "Re-organization" of the National Health Service and there will be difficulty in staffing these committees so that eventually treatment will grind to a halt.

6. There are already arrangements in hand for the improvement of complaints procedures and attention should be drawn to publicity for such arrangements and for the activities of Community Health Councils rather than to set up yet another system.

Appendix VII
FLORIDA GUIDELINES FOR THE USE OF BEHAVIOURAL PROCEDURES IN STATE HOSPITALS FOR THE RETARDED

1. This is the report of a joint task force set up in June, 1974, under the auspices of the Florida Division of Retardation and the Department of Psychology of the Florida State University. Its membership consisted principally of academic and clinical psychologists but also included three lawyers, a Division of Retardation administrator and a representative of the National Association for Retarded Citizens. No general physician or psychiatrist served upon it. The document contains not only the task force report proper but the guidelines based upon it proposed for implementation by the Florida Division of Retardation.

2. After an introductory review of the development of behavioural methods and their applications to the management of retarded (ie mentally handicapped) persons, an account is given of the evolution of existing legal safeguards, and their implications for the conduct of behavioural modification procedures in institutions for the retarded. It is stressed that the inmates of such institutions should be treated as "clients" rather than as "Recipients of aims" and that those who administer programmes designed for their benefit should have clearly defined powers and be accountable for their decisions. Although recognising that a number of procedures employed in psychiatric treatment are potentially open to abuse, the task force limited its inquiry to possible abuse specifically within the sphere of behaviour modification.

3.   A review of behavioural programmes and their organizational contexts is then given and it is pointed out that many of the abuses or misuses of behavioural procedures arise because of lack of competent staff to design and implement them. Recommendations are made regarding the levels of academic qualification and practical experience appropriate to staff at varying levels of responsibility. In particular, it is urged that Directors of Programmes should have a PhD or equivalent degree as well as appropriate experience and be able effectively to coordinate all programmes of behaviour modification in the institution in which they hold office.

4.   The task force further recommend that the Division of Retardation should provide stipends for graduate training of students in mental retardation and applied behaviour analysis and that a State Coordinator of Behavioural Programmes be added to the staff of the Director of the Division in order to expedite the development of in-service training programmes.

5.   It is argued that methods of behaviour modification involve essentially the strengthening of adaptive or 'desirable' behaviour patterns by means of positive reinforcement, with concurrent weakening of maladaptive or 'undesirable' behaviour patterns by means of non-reinforcement ('extinction'). Thus every instance of inappropriate behaviour is ignored while every instance of appropriate behaviour incompatible with it is heavily reinforced. It is argued that the twin processes of reinforcement and extinction provide the essential ingredients of all staff-client interactions in the setting of a behaviour modification programme.

6.   It is the view of the task force that certain procedures which have been demonstrated empirically to weaken a wide range of behaviours must be assessed not only in terms of therapeutic efficacy but also with regard to ethical criteria and public acceptability. Such techniques, which may involve the use of aversive or painful stimuli or the more drastic applications of 'time-out' or seclusion procedures are ordinarily employed only in cases in which the client's behaviour is likely to harm himself or others. Regardless of efficacy, however, such techniques should not be generally used if people believe them to be cruel or inhumane or if they are at all readily subject to abuse by those responsible for their application.

7.   In view of these considerations, the task force make a distinction between techniques of weakening inappropriate behaviour in which the potential for abuse is small or non-existent and those which, in their view, have greater potential for abuse or which have failed to gain full public acceptance. The former include limited use of seclusion ('time-out') procedures, the use of small fines in token economy systems, and guided rehearsal of appropriate activities to weaken those that are inappropriate ('over-correction'). The latter include more drastic physical constraint or seclusion and the use of electric shock as an aversive procedure.

8.   Procedures for advice, review and consent are discussed. The purpose of these procedures is first, to protect the client's welfare and improve the services available to him; secondly, to allow conscientious and well-trained persons to carry out appropriate treatment procedures with a sense of security; and thirdly, to enable the responsible authority (ie the Division of Retardation) to comply as completely as possible with the form and spirit of the requirements established as a result of recent legislation and court decisions.

49

9. To this end, the task force make the following recommendations:

i. The establishment of a small *Peer Review Committee* composed of persons with recognised competence in behaviour programming and modification. This Committee will review and consider procedures proposed for introduction into any institution under the jurisdiction of the Division. It will pay special attention to suggested procedures that fail to comply with the task force's criteria of what may be regarded as standard, reasonable and conventional methods of behaviour modification.

ii. The establishment of a *Committee on Legal and Ethical Protection* for each region of the Division. Each such Committee shall consist of from five to nine members who are not in the employment of the Division and should include an experienced behavioural scientist, a lawyer, and such other persons as may possess a special interest in the rights and welfare of the retarded. It should also include a parent or relative of a retarded person or even a retarded person himself. The functions of this Committee would be to investigate complaints regarding specific behavioural programmes, conduct periodic visitations to institutions responsible to the Division, and assess proposals for new procedures following their approval by the Peer Review Committee. In all cases in which the proposed new procedures fail to comply with the task force's criteria of general acceptability, particular attention would be paid to the issue of informed consent to the treatment, whether obtained from the patient himself or, where necessary, from a parent or guardian.

iii. That the Division promulgates policies and seeks any necessary legislation to indemnify employees who follow the guidelines based on this Report and create appropriate penalties for those who negligently or wilfully fail to follow them.

Appendix VIII
MINNESOTA GUIDELINES FOR BEHAVIOUR MODIFICATION PROGRAMMES

The so-called Minnesota Guidelines went through a number of revisions from 1967 to 1970. The guidelines recognise that behaviour modification techniques represent important additions to available treatment techniques. Like other treatments they are held to be only effective when appropriately prescribed and properly carried out and like other treatments they involve questions concerning patients' rights, dignity and personal integrity. The Guidelines were formulated to provide general orientation and it was felt that they could not cover every situation or substitute for good judgement.

The Guidelines involve carefully drawn definitions of terms. They include a set of general procedural guidelines which maintain that the programme must be completely open to both public and professional scrutiny, subject to requirements of personal privacy, that before behaviour modification treatment patients must be thoroughly assessed in order to establish that the programme would be in the best therapeutic interests of the patients and that where aversive procedures are concerned the patient's consent or the consent of an involved and responsible relative or guardian must be obtained.

Specific procedural guidelines lay down that positive reinforcement procedures must be used where ever possible. Aversive procedures or withdrawal or postponement of positive reinforcement can be introduced only in a context of a positive programme and in particular circumstances, for example the reduction of frequency or elimination of maladaptive behaviour. Any use of time-out procedures must be part of a planned programme and token reinforcement programmes are only permissible when they are based on positive reinforcement systems.

The Guidelines lay down the need for the establishment of Local Review Committees. These are to be established within each Institution by the Medical Services Division and would have the responsibility of obtaining expert help, seeing that each project is devised in such a way that it can be evaluated, obtaining summary progress reports annually and insuring that involved personnel are trained in behaviour modification techniques to be used and updated in this training by in-service training courses. They would also be responsible for ensuring that evaluation of assessment is carried out and that consent procedures are followed. Maintaining the positive nature of the programme as detailed above, would again be the responsibility of the Committee. Certain aspects of the running of programmes would be referred to the Medical Services Division or the Mental Health Policy Committee. These would include reference to the Committee when there is a lack of resolution at a local level about the possible infringement of patients' rights, dignity and physical comfort, when there is proposed use for aversive stimuli and when there are proposals to use more than temporary withdrawal of normally provided goods and services. This latter would include clearance of any token systems when tokens were used to buy any goods or services that the patient would normally be entitled to or have access to.

The main emphases of the Guidelines are on maintenance of positive orientation of the programme, the regular evaluation of the running of the programme, involvement of the Medical Services Division for the types of issue detailed above and the emphasis on training of all hospital personnel who would be involved with the programme. The Guidelines also emphasise the need for inter-institutional meetings.

Appendix IX
LEGAL RESPONSIBILITY

1. Legal responsibility arises either as a result of the terms of a contract or as a general duty of care (tort) or under the provisions of Statutes. Thus, under the National Health Service Act 1946 it is the duty of the Secretary of State to provide the services of specialists and it is the duty of every Executive Council (now replaced by the Family Practitioner Committee) to make arrangements for the provision by medical practitioners of personal medical services. A consultant contracts with the relevant Health Authority (not with the patient) to undertake (inter alia) the diagnosis and treatment of patients and to provide "continuing clinical responsibility for the patients in your charge, allowing for

all proper delegation to, and training of, your staff". The phrase "clinical responsibility" has no legal definition nor is it the equivalent of the legal duty of care.

2.   The 1959 Mental Health Act introduced the term "Responsible Medical Officer", defined as being the medical practitioner in charge of the treatment of a detained patient. The duties of the RMO include the renewal of detention, responsibility for written reports, for granting leave re-classification and restriction of discharge. The term "RMO" is thus only applicable within the context of this Statute and has no legal meaning outside the context of the Act.

3.   A legal duty of care towards patients is owed by each separate individual whether he be a consultant or a porter. Furthermore, the Authority responsible for a hospital is liable in law for the negligence of all its staff who are regarded as servants ("vicarious liability"). The fact that the consultant has contracted with his employer to exercise clinical responsibility for a patient in no way affects or overrides the duty of care owed by say the nurse to that same patient. The required standard of such care varies according to the skills and qualifications of the person—the amount of skill expected of a registrar would be greater than that required of a member of the public but less than would be expected of a consultant. Liability therefore for any mishap will be attributed by the Court to such one or more persons connected with that mishap whom the Court finds have failed to exercise such reasonable degree of care as may be expected, in the circumstances of the case in question, and from such person or persons according to their training and experience. If there has been no such failure then there will be no negligence and so no liability. The Court is not concerned with "accountability" in the managerial sense provided that the consultant in delegating any authority has exercised proper care in so doing.

4.   If there have been several persons whom the Court finds have contributed towards the negligent act then the responsibility for the damage can be apportioned by the Courts among such negligent persons according to the degree of negligence of each of the persons concerned. Responsibility in a case in 1952 was allocated as to 20% on the doctor and 80% on the Hospital Board under the provisions of the Law Reform Act 1935, the Hospital Board having claimed a contribution from the doctor. It would seem quite feasible for a Court to find that any one or more persons being members of a multi-disciplinary team had not exercised a proper degree of their duty of care (in such proportions as decided by the Court) whilst the remaining members were free from criticism and that accordingly any liability for any mishap must fall on the erring members (and vicariously on the employing body) and not on the whole team. Alternatively, the whole team like, for example, a committee authorising a nursing assistant to take a group of patients into town and one patient running away, might be found to be liable for the mishap.

Printed in England for Her Majesty's Stationery Office by Hobbs the Printers of Southampton
(1561) Dd0698218 K16 10/80 G327